END MENTAL HEALTH DISORDERS

WITH VITAMIN THERAPY

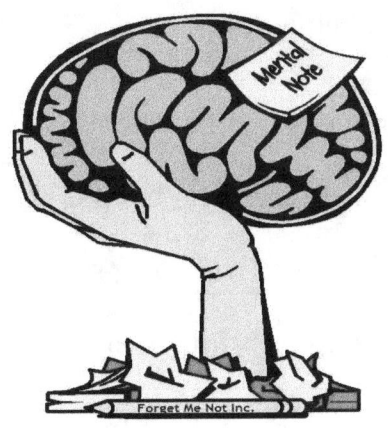

By Patricia A. Carlisle

Introduction

I want to thank you and congratulate you for choosing the book, *"End Mental Health Disorders with Vitamin Therapy"*.

This book contains proven steps and strategies on how to significantly up both your chances in curing your mental health problems, and your defenses against development or worsening of mental illnesses.

This book highlights the significant role of nutrient deficiency in acquirement of a problematic mental health, and the high possibility of winning your fights over such conditions through Vitamin Therapy coupled with practice of healthy diet and lifestyle. Although concrete evidentiary supports for vitamin therapy in the medical arena is in a sense, not fully established as of present, the promising potency of the said program in treatment of modern health issues, not just in the mental aspect that this book focuses on, cannot be disregarded. In fact, as this book will present in the next pages, there are scientific studies that prove the effectiveness of certain vitamins in minimizing, if elimination is not possible at the moment, the harmful effects of common mental conditions such as depression, anxiety, schizophrenia, attention deficit disorder, and cognitive disorders.

Thanks again for choosing this book, I hope you enjoy it!

Table of Contents

Chapter 1

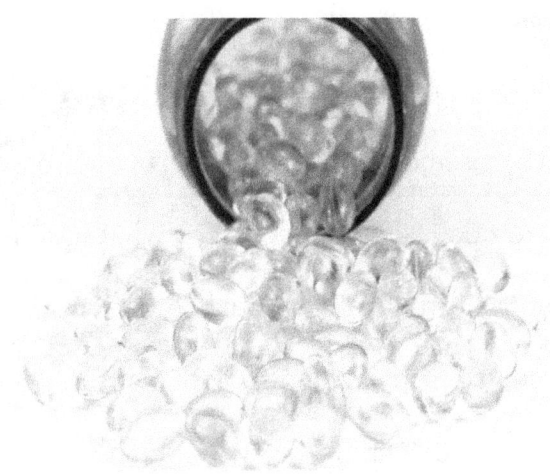

WHAT IS VITAMIN THERAPY?

Vitamin therapy is an emerging type of alternative medicine, specifically of orthomolecular medicine, whose core disease treatment procedure relies on maintenance of health, and correction of the body's biochemical imbalances through optimum nutrition, (i.e. proper and enough attainment of vitamins, minerals, antioxidants, trace elements, amino acids, and essential fatty acids).

Vitamin therapy emphasizes the role of nutrients in prevention of treatment of almost all illnesses, particularly those of degenerative types, such as heart attack, diabetes, cancers, and cognitive deterioration. Vitamin therapy is done by nutrient supplementation or diet programs, or both. Depending on the disease, and specific nutrient deficiency that is scientifically linked to the said disease, an expert can advise which type of vitamins to take as supplement, (or what food to regularly take to get the required nutrient) to the patient. For example, if the patient suffers from depression, he/she may undergo diagnostic tests for vitamin B deficiency, and correspondingly be prescribed with vitamin B-rich supplements and dietary practice. More of this shall be discussed on the next chapters.

Chapter 2

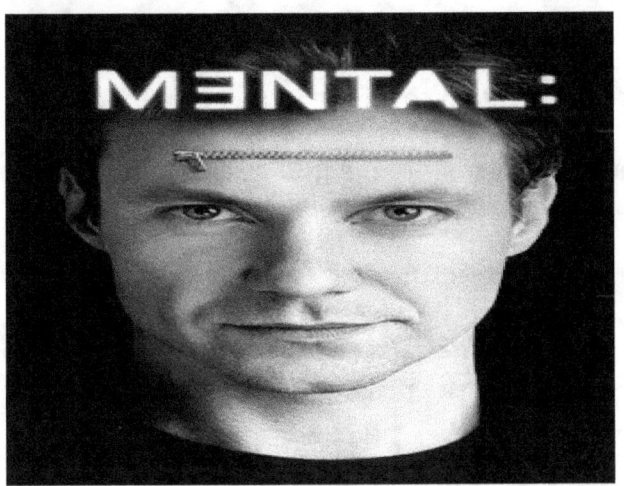

MENTAL HEALTH AND VITAMIN THERAPY

"The mind and the body are separate entities" – this is the common, yet unstated assumption, of majority of conventional methods of disease treatment. If you suffer from a kidney disease, most likely, your doctor will prescribe you with a drug and procedures (dialysis, surgery, etc.) that will directly target the kidneys, and the debilitating manifestations of such condition, including pain and urination problems.

Vitamin therapy believes otherwise. Like most alternative medicines today, vitamin therapy underlines the fact that is being supported by modern science only now, which is the concept of holism. The mind and the body is a holistic composition of biochemical, metabolic, and hormonal operations that are interlinked together in a complex web. In a similar way, a human body's organs and systems, no matter the large difference of their physical distance with each other, and the nature of their physiology, interact and effectively function as one entity. A sickness or health of the body significantly affects the mind or mental health as well. Likewise, a sickness or health of the mind can manifest biologically in organs or systems.

Treating mental disorders with supplements and proper nutrition, in its own, makes sense, either you're an expert or not. It is the micronutrients which construct and maintain the brain's normal architecture, and fuel the organ's biochemical constituents and processes. Micronutrients help build Vitamins, minerals, and other nutrients are just as crucial to other organs of the body. According to biochemist Bruce Ames of the Children's Hospital Oakland Research Institute, not having the right amounts of the 40 micronutrients that a normal human body needs is enough to destroy our biochemistry at a cellular level.

The effectiveness of vitamin therapy in treatment of mental illnesses, as well as most alternative medicines that use natural herbs and food supplementation, relies on its capability to target biochemical and metabolic pathways of organs, and in some cases, boost neural and hormonal activities. For instance, St. John's Wort, a flowering plant, is known to effectively subdue depression symptoms by enhancing the activity of neurotransmitters, particularly norepinephrine and serotonin.

Biochemical's, hormones and metabolic functions have greater roles at play in mental health conditions, and cognitive disorders than what we and medical experts previously believed. Almost of all these factors are derived, processed and/or influenced by what our bodies absorb from the things we put in our mouths. Vitamin therapy exploits this natural truth of the human body. Macronutrients, vitamins, minerals, trace elements, antioxidants and fatty acids, which we acquire from the food we eat or fluids we drink, are essential in maintaining the regular functions of our body at a cellular level, and preventing any abnormality, which can lead to diseases, from happening. Vitamin therapy emphasizes the potency of such nutrients in treatment of diseases.

Vitamin therapy is not just for the treatment of biological diseases, and the maintenance of physical health. In fact, as this book discusses, mental health can be greatly improved by vitamin therapy, and studies support the significant role of such therapy in treating mental illnesses.

Chapter 3

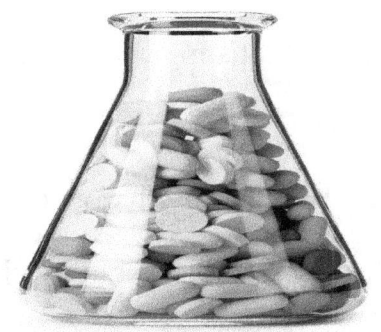

PROMISING POTENCY OF VITAMINS IN COMMON MENTAL HEALTH CONDITIONS

In the late 90s, Bernard Gesch, an Oxford University physiologist, conducted a study that used 231 prisoners as test subjects. The test subjects were divided into 2 groups. The first group was given the recommended vitamins and minerals, as well as supplements of fish oil and evening primrose daily. The second group on the other hand was given placebos daily. The test subjects were monitored for almost a year. The results recorded found an almost 35% decrease in antisocial acts committed by the first group compared to the second one. A significant reduction in violent incidents was also reported by the prison warden, few weeks after the commencement of the said study.

This is just one of the many studies that support the significant role of proper nutrition in moods, emotions, social behaviors, and overall mental health. For more than 60 years, conventional medicine, specifically psychology and psychiatry, ignored and even refused to believe the benefits of nutrients such as vitamins and minerals in maintaining health in both physical and mental contexts. Chapters 3 and 4 shall discuss the effectiveness of certain vitamins in treatment of the most common mental health conditions that are backed by scientific studies. Recommendations for dietary habits and lifestyle shall also be provided in the said chapters.

Depression and Anxiety

Depression and anxiety are two of the most common mental health conditions that afflict people today. Genetics, social and personal issues, environmental agents, stress, and other diseases are generally the factors that were considered by experts before to trigger the said conditions. Recent studies however are shedding light to the biochemical nature of these mental conditions, and likewise the potential that use of biochemistry in treating them poses, particularly in the aspects of food and diet.

In some studies, a deficiency in B vitamins was found to play a role in the development of depression and anxiety. B vitamins are known key players in the brain's enzymatic processes, and biochemical pathways. For instance, most B vitamins, particularly Vitamin B-12, produce biochemical's that significantly affect certain brain functions, such as moods. Vitamin B1 participates in regulation of blood sugar, while Vitamin B3 or niacin is involved in the synthesis of serotonin, a neurotransmitter. Recent studies have linked low levels of serotonin to development of mild to severe cases of depression, anxiety, and other mood disorders. A dose of 1000-3000 mg of Vitamin B3 daily is enough to risks of developing or worsening anxiety.

Vitamin B3 also possesses more powerful resistance against free radicals, which are primary progenitors of degenerative diseases of this generation, especially if taken along with vitamin E and C, and trace element selenium. The nutritive potency of Vitamin B3 is quite indispensable, that it has been one of the primary nutrients likely used in Mega-vitamin Therapy.

Another B vitamin that's potent against depression is Vitamin B6. Vitamin B5 has been found to be effective on adrenal operations and regulation of stress, which is one of the leading causes of depression.

Vitamin D, a fat-soluble vitamin and hormone which is crucial to maintaining immune, bone, heart and muscle health, was also found to have a relevant effect on depression and anxiety. In one study, Vitamin D deficiency was found to cause depression in patients with fibromyalgia. The similar association of minor to severe cases of depressions to Vitamin D deficiency was also concluded by research studies conducted in Netherlands and the UK. This correlation was observed more on people aged 65 years and older.

Although experts are still unsuccessful in grasping the real deal about the link between depression and Vitamin D, similar studies to those which were previously mentioned are more than enough to convince them that Vitamin D is indeed a key player in depression pathophysiology and treatment. Aside from its famous supporting role to calcium absorption,

Vitamin D has receptors all throughout the brain, where it helps in the production of neurotransmitters.

Alcoholism

In 1960, Abram Hoffer, together with Alcoholics Anonymous' founder Bill Wilson (or Bill W. as he's famously called), witnessed the healing potential of Mega-vitamin Therapy. The said therapy involved a daily intake of 3000-mg Vitamin B3. Bill W. reported disappearance of fatigue and depression which had afflicted him for years, just after a few weeks of the therapy. He recommended this to his peers in AA and the results were the same. Although doctors are still skeptical about Vitamin B3's wondrous effects in dealing with alcoholism, and other mental conditions that come with it, including depression, anxiety and schizophrenia, both clinical and anecdotal evidences are still too difficult to ignore, or be considered as baseless.

Schizophrenia

Most patients suffering from schizophrenia, particularly those of the male sex were found to have high levels of homocysteine in the blood. Homocysteine is a toxic amino acid that interferes with the body's methylation process, or the process of regulating chemical balance. It is processed by the body from digested protein. The only way to mitigate such increase in homocysteine levels is by getting B vitamins, especially Vitamin B12, Vitamin B6 and folic.

High levels of homocysteine can still be present among people who don't show any lack of vitamins whatsoever. This condition doesn't appear to be connected to any dietary or lifestyle choices, like smoking, either. Experts believe that such cases are the result of genetic makeup, wherein the patient is born with an abnormal homocysteine-lowering enzyme. The need for more vitamins and other nutrients that regulate homocysteine levels in the blood is therefore greater for schizophrenic patients who possess this kind of genetic anomaly.

Fatty acids are also essential to brain's overall health of patients suffering from schizophrenia. Essential fatty acids such as Omega-3, Omega-6 and Omega-9, inhibits oxidation, which is facilitated by oxidants that we usually get from unhealthy food (especially fried or charred) and lifestyle habits (e.g. smoking). These fatty acids make the bioavailability, or the ease of absorption by the body, easier for antioxidants, such as vitamins A, C and E. Vitamin C, due to its immune-boosting prowess, is also important to maintaining the health of schizophrenics. This vitamin is also a powerful stress-reducer that counters excessive adrenaline, which is very common in patients suffering from schizophrenia.

Bipolar Disorder

There are clinical evidences that support the potency of B vitamins in treating bipolar disorder. Low levels of folic acid and Vitamin B-12 are linked to triggering manic episodes.

Although this claim needs more research to become established as a fact, the role of Vitamin B-12 in the production of dopamine, serotonin, and other mood-regulating biochemical's in the brain remains unchallenged.

Folic acid can enhance the effectiveness of lithium, one of the most prescribed drugs to people with bipolar disorder. Choline and inositol, compounds that are classified as B-complex vitamins, also showed potential in reducing symptoms of bipolar disorder.

Recommendations:

Vitamin deficiency can result from poor dietary choices, and malabsorption of nutrients by the body. B vitamins, particularly the most potent types, are abundant in animal products, such as fish, shellfish, lean meat, eggs, and dairy products. These nutrients cannot be found in plant foods, that's why quite a number of people who have B vitamin deficiency are vegans or vegetarians. Malabsorption on the other hand, can be a result of either a digestive disease or genetics. Vitamin D can also be obtained from fatty fishes (mackerel, cod), meat and early morning sunlight. Fruits and vegetables are rich in Vitamins A, C and E.

People with digestive illnesses such as Crohn's disease, or celiac disease have minimally effective small intestines, which makes it difficult to absorb nutrients from digested food. There are also people who were naturally born with nutrient malabsorption problems. In any case, the need to alter food choices, lifestyle habits, and food supplementation is greater for such people. Consulting with a medical expert to determine if you have nutrient deficiency, and the possible anomalies in your body which caused this deficiency is recommended. Regular intake of animal-based foods at appropriate amounts must be practiced. Supplementation of vitamins with an amount of at least 10 times the recommended dietary allowance is also important, as reported by a neuropsychobiological study, which found significant improvement in mood in both genders in just 3 months of vitamin intake.

Chapter 4

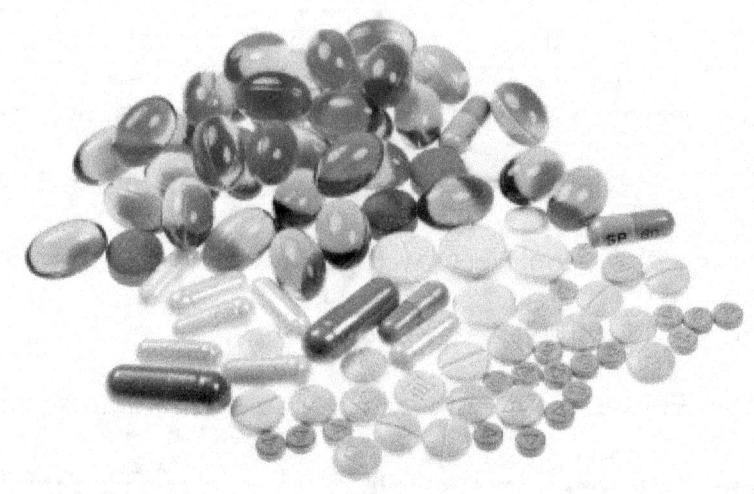

Role of Vitamins against Cognitive Deterioration

In the previous chapter, the connection between B vitamin deficiency and common mental illnesses such as depression, anxiety, and schizophrenia is introduced and discussed. If you're still unconvinced on the seriousness of this nutrient's deficiency poses to one's body, and quality of life, then this Chapter might make you think otherwise. Deficiency- in essential vitamins not only predisposes yourself to the risk of the aforementioned mental illnesses. It can also expose you to the susceptibility of developing cognitive deterioration later in life, and the indicative signs of such scenario show themselves even at ages as young as 8 – 10 years old.

Dementia and Alzheimer's disease

Vitamin B3 or niacin deficiency can cause a disease called *pellagra*. This disease is characterized by 3 primary manifestations, mainly: diarrhea, dermatitis, and dementia. Other symptoms include sleep apnea, depression and anxiety, headaches and thought disorder.

Deficiency in Vitamin B12 on the other hand can lead to a rare condition called *pernicious anemia*, which is characterized by formation larger yet fewer red blood cells in the bone marrow. Its symptoms include jaundice, fatigue and lethargy, headaches, breathing difficulty, numbness, or tingling (especially in the hands and feet), and trouble with keeping balance. Other symptoms which are commonly observed in older people include slowness, mood swings, irritability, confusion, and apathy. Pernicious anemia is also blamed for the development of some dementia cases.

There are also several studies which show the possible link between developing dementia and Alzheimer's diseases, and deficiency in Vitamin D.

Memory Loss and Cognitive Decline

Researchers found that Vitamin B-12 deficiency is strongly associated to thinking problems, memory loss and brain shrinkage. Low levels of Vitamin B-12 have been observed to be common in almost 40% of the elderly population aged 60 years or more. Scientists think that some of the symptoms commonly associated to aging, such as memory loss, slow reflexes, and overall cognitive degeneration, are possibly attributed to decreased levels of Vitamin B-12.

The Tufts University Framingham Offspring Study however, found that Vitamin B-12 deficiency afflicts young people as much as it does old people. Another study concluded that Vitamin B-12 deficiency also occurs in kids who particularly practiced a vegan diet until the age of six. These kids showed lower scores in fluid intelligence, which involves reasoning, problem-solving, abstract thinking, and learning skills, compared to their peers who have practiced a regular diet. They also scored lower in terms of memory and spatial ability. The same findings were observed years after the same kids began to include meat-based food in their diet. The results are quite alarming, according to experts, since these can have irreversible consequences in the kids' individual functioning.

Vitamin B-12, together with foliate, plays a significant role in DNA synthesis, and production of red blood cells. It is also crucial in building and maintenance of the brain's myelin sheath, a protective layer that surrounds the nerves. This insulating layer also promotes fast and easy transmission of impulses among neurons. Any deficiency in the said vitamin can pose degenerative risks to a person's brain and cognitive skills.

Recommendations:

Cobalamin or Vitamin B-12 is the sole vitamin that possesses cobalt, a trace element (hence the name). Plants have no use for this element, so they don't store it. Cobalamin can only be produced in animals, especially in their gut. It is abundant in eggs, meat, seafood's and dairy products, and is easily absorbed, and stored in the liver.

For people who still have problems with cobalamin deficiency despite the inclusion of cobalamin-rich foods in their diet, there is the choice of supplementation, and recently, cobalamin injections. Vitamin B-12 or Cobalamin injections were especially created for patients who suffer from serious conditions like pernicious anemia, and yet are unable to properly absorb the nutrient through food consumption due to genetic factors, or inflammatory gut illnesses. Cobalamin also has forms that can be taken orally or nasally.

The most frequently used forms of Vitamin B-12 are cyanocobalamin, methylcobalamin, and hydroxycobalamin, which are specially administered for patients with neurological impairments.

Clinical trials found that administration of Vitamin B-12 on patients with dementia at a designed timing window prior to the onset of the disease's first manifestations, can delay its development.

Studies also found that taking 2,000 - 5,000 IU of Vitamin D every day is enough to counter Vitamin D deficiency. Some doctors usually prescribe a dosage of 50,000 IU of Vitamin D per week, until such time that the patient reaches the desired levels of Vitamin D. When choosing Vitamin D supplements, select Vitamin D3 or cholecalciferol, which is the most effective form of Vitamin D, and take this with a large meal.

Chapter 5

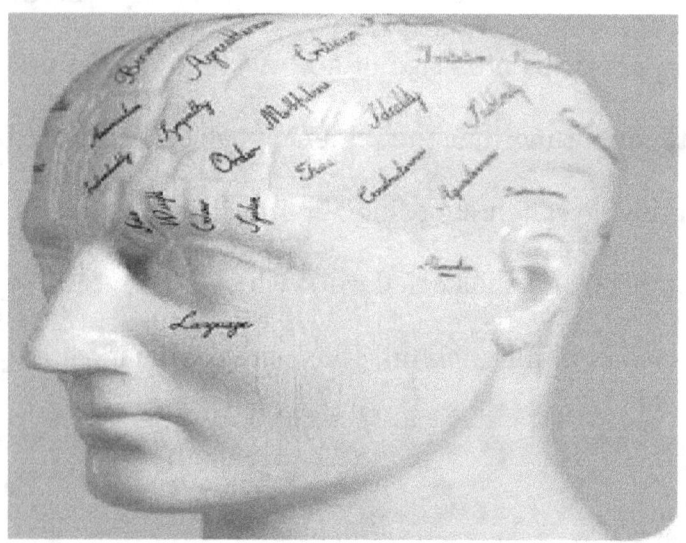

OTHER NUTRIENT HEROES FOR MENTAL HEALTH AND WELLNESS

Vitamins are not the only nutrients that we need to combat mental health disorders, or any kind of disease for that matter. The body also needs minerals, antioxidants, essential fatty acids, and trace elements on a daily basis, to ensure overall health and protection from free radicals, and disease agents. These nutrients include magnesium, calcium, zinc, iron, iodine, selenium, Omega 3 and 6 fatty acids, and amino acids, among others.

Magnesium

Magnesium is crucial to the nourishment of the central nervous system, as well as the cardiovascular system. Studies found that together with Vitamin B-6, magnesium can reduce, or prevent nervousness, panic attacks, irritability, restlessness and fear in patients afflicted with anxiety. If taken with calcium, magnesium can promote proper and stress-free sleep. The typical daily recommendation for magnesium is 400 – 600mg. Magnesium is also abundant in dark green vegetables, such as kale, chard, mustard greens and spinach, as well as seafood's, poultry meat, beef, legumes, nuts and seeds, potatoes and fruits like figs and watermelons. Quinoa, buckwheat, oats, millet, and other unrefined grains are a rich source of both B vitamins and magnesium. Spices like peppermint and sage are also rich in magnesium.

Essential Fatty Acids

Essential fatty acids such as Omega 3 and Omega 6 have been the subject of many studies that aim to understand the pathophysiology of mental and cognitive disorders, and discover their possible treatments. There are some researches which claim that a significant reduction in anger and anxiety were found in substance abusers who have been given fish oil as food supplement for 3 months. These fatty acids are also linked to cognitive improvement. In Iceland where fish is a staple food, most women were found to have given birth to babies with larger brain mass. Omega 3 is abundant in fish meat and other fish products, while Omega 6 is plentiful in evening primrose oil.

Amino Acids

Amino acids such as L-thiamine and Lactium have been found to reduce stress-related symptoms, as well as anxiety and depression. The former also produces a calming effect by increasing the levels of GABA neurotransmitter.

Chromium

There are several studies that linked chromium picolinate to alleviation of depression, and even improve a patient's response to ADDs (antidepressant drugs).

Iodine

Iodine, which is abundant in seafood's such as shellfish and seaweeds, is crucial to brain functions due to its important role in metabolic activities of cerebral cells. Deficiency in iodine can also cause a significant decrease in learning skills and intelligence, especially among children.

Iron

Iron is essential to oxygenation of the blood. It is also crucial in synthesis of neurotransmitters and building of myelin sheath. Studies found that infantile anemia, or the anemic condition that affects very young children with iron deficiency, can significantly interferes with cognitive development. Iron also produces positive effects on patients with depression.

Selenium

According to studies, deficiency in selenium is associated with anxiety symptoms, and mood swings.

Zinc

Zinc is essential in protecting the cells from damages, and degeneration caused by free radicals. This element is particularly important in maintenance of the immune system. There are also clinical studies which found the effectiveness of oral zinc supplements in suppressing depression

Chapter 6

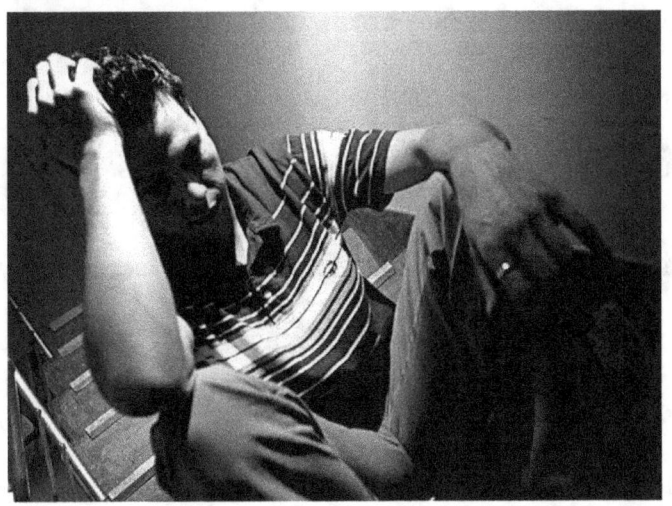

ADDITIONAL ALTERNATIVE METHODS OF TREATMENT

Based on the discussions made in the previous chapters, Vitamin Therapy is not just a quack alternative for treatment of mental disorders. Indeed, nutrition is always the best weapon any kind of disease, and Vitamin Therapy emphasizes this fact. However, diseases, particularly those that involve mental health, possess myriad causes, and one treatment method cannot always work on its own. Medical experts today are open-minded enough to consider, or even embrace, the health benefits of alternative methods of disease treatment, but still, if we are not to take care of our body, there will still be negative consequences of our wrong health choices, despite the availability, or use of conventional drugs, medical technologies and yes, alternative medicine procedures.

For instance, it is important to be physically active as regularly as possible. Our bodies are like machines which are predisposed to damage, wearing and breakage if not operated, and maintained regularly. Regular exercise, that means at least an hour of physical activity, 3 times a week, can flush out toxins, improve metabolism, and respiration, enhance heart endurance, remove stress, increase oxygen intake, and even help with depression and anxiety.

Meditation and stress-management therapies are what we call mind exercises. These can significantly reduce depression symptoms, and remove stress as well. It also improves concentration, memory, and cognitive abilities.

Conclusion

Thank you again for choosing this book!

I hope this book was able to help you to understand how Vitamin therapy works, and the wonders it can do in dealing and managing your health problems, particularly those of mental aspect. Although there are research and evidences that can back the effectiveness of Vitamin therapy, it is still largely outside the established boundaries of conventional medicine. Doctors indeed recognize the beneficial use of nutritional programs such as, Vitamin therapy in treatment of diseases, but the fact that there are some studies which concluded either the non-efficacy, or toxicity of some vitamins and minerals (particularly in large doses) still exist.

Moreover, we cannot deny the fact that diseases on their own still have secrets hidden away from the prying eyes of advanced medical technology. There are myriad of causes of diseases, and based on what we see in the news and results of medical studies, the conventional practice of one drug equals one medical symptom isn't as effective as we previously believe. That's why consulting with an expert first to treat your conditions before trying anything new is strictly recommended. The need for more research to shed light on these inconsistencies is therefore crucial, particularly in this generation wherein people of all age, and ethnicity is continuously threatened by serious degenerative illnesses.

The next step is to consult with your doctor, dietitian and nutritionist about the status of your mental health, and the possible nutrient deficiency that your body is currently experiencing. Vitamin therapy might be just the thing you've been waiting for to finally change the way you're living your life, for the better. Vitamin Therapy, like most non-conventional treatment procedures, is based on holism, i.e. the health of the each part is the health of the whole. Overall health and wellness, and resistance against any type of disease, can only be achieved if the body acquires appropriate amount of nutrients (vitamins, minerals and antioxidants) every day, and regular exercise is practiced. You shouldn't eliminate as well the importance of conventional medicine and other alternative treatment procedures, such as stress management programs and cognitive behavior therapy, in treating mental health conditions.

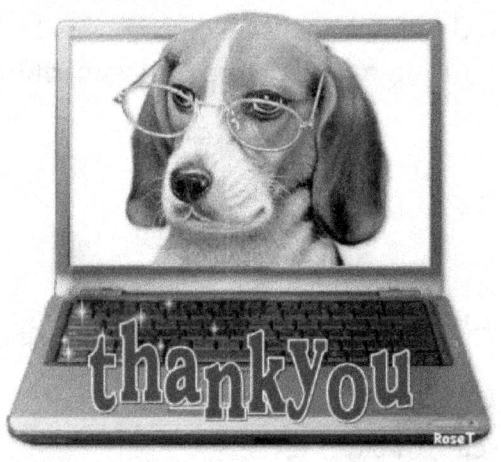

If you enjoyed this book, please take the time to share your thoughts and post a review on Amazon. It'd be greatly appreciated!

Thank you and good luck!

Preview Of 'Juicing to Help Mental Illness: Awesome juicing recipes for a healthier mental health.'

Mental illness is becoming more and more common in today's world, and most of the times unrecognized, the cause of this may be simple nutrient deficiency. If not addressed, mental illnesses cause by nutrient deficiency can take a serious toll on our physical and mental health, which is why it is important to correct it early through juicing and other nutritional means.

Chapter 1

Berry A-Peeling

Ingredients

Apples-2 large (3-1/4" dia)

Lime-1/2 fruit (2" dia)

Strawberries-3 cup, whole

Directions: Process all ingredients in a juicer, shaker or stir and serve

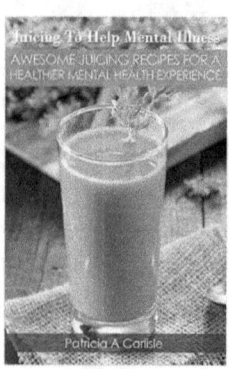

CHECK OUT THE REST OF (JUICING TO HELP MENTAL ILLNESS: AWESOME JUICING RECIPES FOR A HEALTHIER MENTAL HEALTH) ON AMAZON.

Check Out My Other Books

Below you'll find some of my other popular books that are popular on Amazon and Kindle as well. Alternatively, you can visit my author page on Amazon to see other work done by me.

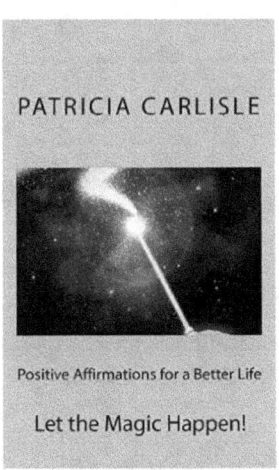

POSITIVE AFFIRMATIONS FOR A BETTER LIFE.

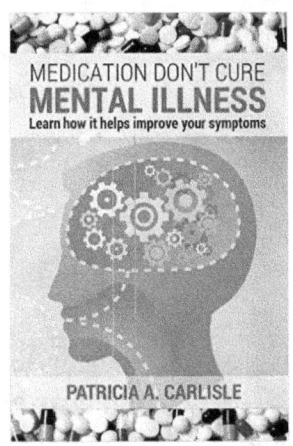

MEDICATION DON'T CURE MENTAL ILLNESS:
Learn how to it helps improve your symptoms.

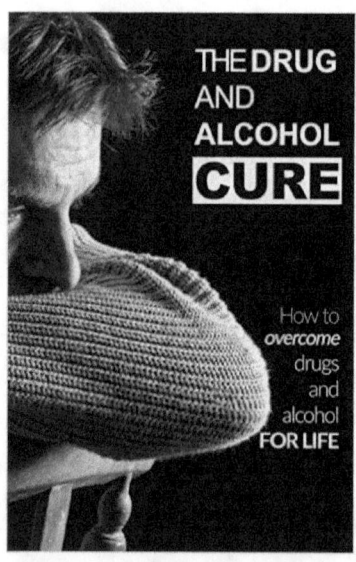

THE DRUG AND ALCOHOL CURE: How to overcome drugs and alcohol for life.

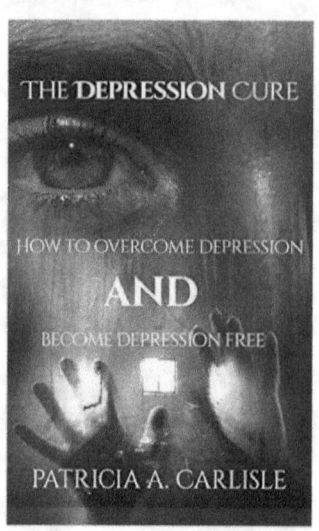

THE DEPRESSION CURE: How to overcome depression and become depression free.

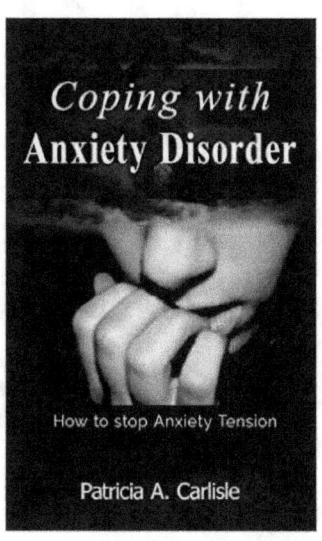

COPING WITH ANXIETY DISORDER: How to stop Anxiety Tension.

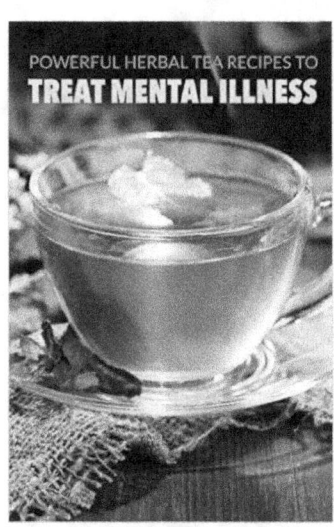

POWERFUL HERBAL RECIPES TO TREAT MENTAL ILLNESS.

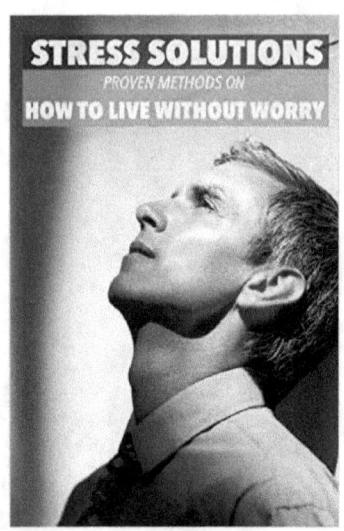

STRESS SOLUTIONS: Proven methods on how to live without worry.

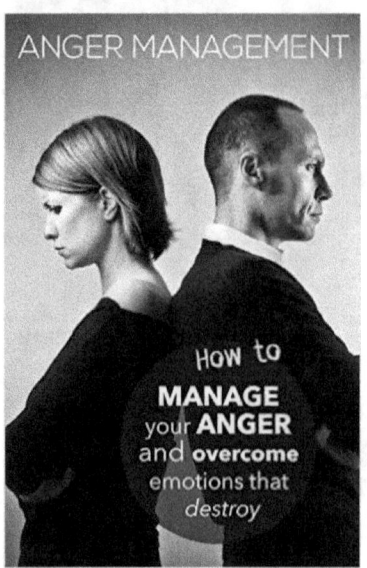

ANGER MANAGEMENT: How to manage your anger and overcome emotions that destroy.

BONUS: SUBSCRIBE TO THE FREE BOOK

Beginners Guide to Yoga & Meditation

"Stressed out? Do You Feel Like The World Is Crashing Down Around You? Want To Take A Vacation That Will Relax Your Mind, Body And Spirit? Well this Easy To Read Step By Step

E-Book Makes It All Possible!"

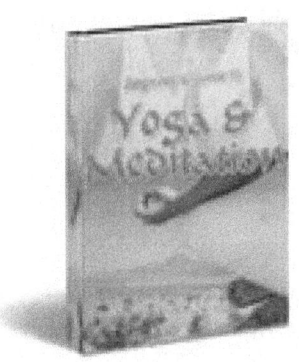

Instructions on how to join our mailing list, and receive a free copy of "Yoga and Meditation" can be found in any of my Kindle eBooks.

NOTES

NOTES

NOTES

NOTES

NOTES

NOTES

NOTES